CONTENTS

INTRODUCTION

Explanation Of Endomorph Body Type And Its Impact On Weight Loss And Muscle Building

The endomorph body type is one of the three basic somatotypes, which are a classification system used to describe body types. Endomorphs are generally characterized by a larger frame, with a tendency to store more fat and a slower metabolism. They may also have shorter limbs and a rounder body shape.

The impact of the endomorph body type on weight loss and muscle building can be significant. Endomorphs may find it more difficult to lose weight and build muscle compared to other body types due to their slower metabolism and tendency to store fat. However, with the right nutrition plan and exercise regimen, endomorphs can still achieve their fitness goals.

The endomorph diet takes into account the unique nutritional needs of endomorphs, with a focus on balancing macronutrients to support weight loss and muscle building. Endomorphs may need to pay particular attention to their carbohydrate intake, as they may be more prone to insulin resistance, which can lead to weight gain.

In terms of exercise, endomorphs may benefit from a combination of cardiovascular exercise and strength training to boost their metabolism and build lean muscle mass. It's important for endomorphs to find an exercise routine that they enjoy and can stick to in the long term.

By understanding the impact of their body type on weight loss and muscle building, endomorphs can tailor their diet and exercise regimen to achieve their fitness goals.

Importance Of Nutrition For Achieving Fitness Goals

Nutrition is a crucial component of achieving fitness goals. A healthy, well-balanced diet provides the necessary fuel and nutrients for the body to function optimally during physical activity. It also supports muscle growth and recovery after exercise.

Proper nutrition can also help with weight management. Consuming more calories than the body needs can lead to weight gain, while consuming fewer calories than the body needs can lead to weight loss. By eating the right amount of calories and balancing macronutrients (carbohydrates, protein, and fat), individuals can achieve their desired weight and body composition.

In addition, nutrition can impact athletic performance. Adequate hydration, proper fueling before exercise, and replenishing nutrients after exercise can all improve endurance, strength, and recovery time.

The importance of nutrition is especially relevant for individuals with specific fitness goals, such as building muscle, losing weight, or improving athletic performance. In these cases, a customized nutrition plan may be necessary to support these goals.

Overall, nutrition plays a critical role in achieving fitness goals. A healthy, well-balanced diet that supports physical activity can help individuals reach their desired weight, body composition, and athletic performance.

Overview Of The Endomorph Diet And Its Principles

The endomorph diet is a nutrition plan that is designed to help individuals with an endomorph body type reach their fitness goals. Endomorphs tend to have a slower metabolism and store more fat, so the diet focuses on balancing macronutrients to promote weight loss and muscle building.

The principles of the endomorph diet include:

1. **Balancing macronutrients:** The endomorph diet emphasizes a balance of carbohydrates, protein, and fat to support weight loss and muscle building. Endomorphs may need to pay particular attention to their carbohydrate intake and choose complex carbohydrates over simple sugars.

2. **Adequate protein intake:** Protein is essential for building and repairing muscle tissue. Endomorphs may benefit from consuming

protein-rich foods such as lean meats, fish, and legumes to support muscle growth.

3. **Healthy fats:** Healthy fats are an important component of the endomorph diet as they can help regulate hormone production and reduce inflammation. Endomorphs may benefit from consuming sources of healthy fats such as avocado, nuts, and olive oil.

4. **Managing calorie intake:** Endomorphs may be prone to weight gain, so managing calorie intake is essential. The endomorph diet recommends eating frequent, smaller meals throughout the day to maintain energy levels and prevent overeating.

5. **Hydration:** Adequate hydration is crucial for overall health and athletic performance. The endomorph diet recommends drinking plenty of water throughout the day and avoiding sugary drinks.

By following the principles of the endomorph diet, individuals can support their weight loss and muscle building goals. It's important to work with a qualified healthcare provider or nutritionist to develop a customized plan that meets individual needs and goals.

CHAPTER ONE

Understanding Endomorphs And Their Unique Nutritional Needs

Endomorphs are individuals with a particular body type characterized by a larger frame, higher body fat percentage, and slower metabolism. Their unique body type makes them more prone to storing fat and gaining weight, and it can also impact their nutritional needs.

To support their weight loss and muscle-building goals, endomorphs have specific nutritional needs. Here are a few considerations for an endomorph diet:

1. **Balance macronutrients:** Endomorphs should focus on balancing macronutrients (carbohydrates, protein, and fat) to support weight loss and muscle building. A balanced diet will help stabilize blood sugar and insulin levels, which can be important for endomorphs who may be more prone to insulin resistance.

2. **Manage carbohydrates:** Endomorphs may need to manage their carbohydrate intake more closely than other body types. Carbohydrates can be an important energy source during

exercise, but too many can lead to weight gain. Endomorphs may need to choose complex carbohydrates over simple sugars and may benefit from eating carbohydrates in smaller, more frequent meals.

3. **Consume adequate protein:** Protein is essential for muscle growth and repair. Endomorphs may need to consume more protein than other body types to support their muscle-building goals. Lean meats, fish, and legumes are all good sources of protein.

4. **Incorporate healthy fats:** Endomorphs should incorporate healthy fats into their diet. Healthy fats can help regulate hormone production, reduce inflammation, and support overall health. Sources of healthy fats include nuts, seeds, avocado, and olive oil.

5. **Stay hydrated:** Adequate hydration is important for overall health and athletic performance. Endomorphs should drink plenty of water throughout the day and avoid sugary drinks that can contribute to weight gain.

By understanding their unique nutritional needs, endomorphs can develop a diet plan that supports their fitness goals and helps them achieve optimal health. It's important to work with a qualified healthcare provider or nutritionist to develop a customized plan that meets individual needs and goals.

Detailed Description Of Endomorph Body Type

The human body is not a one-size-fits-all model, and individuals differ in their body composition, which is often determined by genetics. Endomorphs are one of the three main body types, along with ectomorphs and mesomorphs. Endomorphs typically have a larger, rounder body shape, with a higher percentage of body fat compared to muscle mass. They may have a slower metabolism, making it easier for them to gain weight and harder for them to lose it. Endomorphs typically have a softer, curvier appearance, with a tendency to store fat in the hips, thighs, and buttocks.

Endomorphs are often described as having a "pear-shaped" body type, with a larger lower body and smaller upper body. This body type is often associated with a shorter, more compact frame, with a broader waistline and wider hips. Endomorphs typically have a slower metabolism, making it easier for them to gain weight and harder for them to lose it. This is because their bodies are more efficient at storing fat, and they may have a tendency to overeat or consume more calories than their body needs.

Despite these challenges, endomorphs can still achieve a healthy and fit body. Regular exercise, a balanced diet, and a healthy lifestyle can help to improve metabolism and promote weight loss. Endomorphs may benefit from incorporating resistance training into their workout routine, as this can help to build muscle and boost metabolism. It is also important for endomorphs to pay attention to their nutrition and choose foods that are nutrient-dense and low in calories.

How Metabolism Works In Endomorphs

Metabolism refers to the chemical processes that occur within the body to convert food into energy. Endomorphs may have a slower metabolism compared to other body types, making it more difficult for them to lose weight. This is because their bodies are more efficient at storing fat, and they may have a tendency to overeat or consume more calories than their body needs.

One way to improve metabolism is to engage in regular

exercise. This can help to increase muscle mass, which can boost metabolism and promote weight loss. Endomorphs may benefit from incorporating both cardio and resistance training into their workout routine, as this can help to burn calories and build muscle.

Another way to improve metabolism is to eat a healthy and balanced diet. Endomorphs may benefit from focusing on nutrient-dense foods that are low in calories, such as fruits, vegetables, lean protein, and whole grains. It is also important to avoid consuming too many sugary or processed foods, which can lead to weight gain and negatively impact metabolism.

Finally, endomorphs may benefit from getting enough sleep and managing stress levels. Sleep deprivation and stress can both negatively impact metabolism, making it more difficult to lose weight. Prioritizing sleep and stress management can help to improve overall health and promote weight loss.

Nutritional Requirements For Endomorphs

Endomorphs may have a slower metabolism, making it

more difficult for them to lose weight. However, with the right nutrition, endomorphs can still achieve a healthy and fit body. Here are some key nutritional requirements for endomorphs:

1. **Caloric intake:** Endomorphs may need to consume fewer calories than other body types in order to lose weight. However, it is important to make sure that they are still consuming enough calories to support their overall health and energy levels. Consulting with a registered dietitian can help endomorphs determine their optimal caloric intake.

2. **Macronutrient balance:** Endomorphs may benefit from focusing on a balanced diet that includes a combination of carbohydrates, proteins, and healthy fats. Carbohydrates provide energy for the body, while proteins help to build and maintain muscle mass. Healthy fats, such as those found in nuts, seeds, and avocados, can help to promote satiety and support overall health.

3. **Fiber:** Endomorphs may benefit from consuming a diet high in fiber. Fiber can help to promote satiety and regulate blood sugar levels, which can help to prevent overeating and weight gain. Good sources of fiber include fruits, vegetables, whole grains, and legumes.

4. **Hydration:** Staying hydrated is important for

all body types, but it is especially important for endomorphs. Drinking enough water can help to regulate appetite, support digestion, and promote overall health. Endomorphs should aim to drink at least 8-10 glasses of water per day.

5. **Vitamins and minerals:** Endomorphs may be at risk for nutrient deficiencies if they are not consuming a balanced diet. It is important to consume a variety of nutrient-dense foods to ensure that they are getting all of the vitamins and minerals that their body needs. Consulting with a registered dietitian can help endomorphs determine if they need to supplement their diet with any vitamins or minerals.

In conclusion, endomorphs have a unique body type that can make it more difficult to lose weight. However, with the right nutrition and lifestyle choices, endomorphs can still achieve a healthy and fit body. Regular exercise, a balanced diet, and a healthy lifestyle are all key to improving metabolism and promoting weight loss in endomorphs.

CHAPTER TWO
THE SCIENCE BEHIND THE ENDOMORPH DIET

Explanation Of Macronutrients And Their Importance In The Diet

Macronutrients are nutrients that the body requires in large amounts to function properly. They are the building blocks of a healthy diet and provide energy, promote growth and repair of tissues, and maintain bodily functions. There are three primary macronutrients: carbohydrates, proteins, and fats.

Carbohydrates are the body's primary source of energy. They are broken down into glucose and used by cells for fuel. Carbohydrates are found in foods such as bread, pasta, rice, fruits, and vegetables. There are two types of carbohydrates: simple and complex. Simple carbohydrates, such as those found in candy and sugary drinks, are quickly digested and provide a rapid burst of energy. Complex carbohydrates, such as those found in whole grains and vegetables, take longer to digest and provide sustained energy.

Proteins are important for growth and repair of tissues. They are made up of amino acids, which are essential for the body to function properly. Protein is found in foods such as meat, poultry, fish, beans, and nuts. It is important to consume a variety of protein sources to ensure that the body gets all of the necessary amino acids.

Fats are essential for the absorption of certain vitamins and minerals and for the production of hormones. They are also a source of energy for the body. Fats can be found in foods such as nuts, seeds, oils, and fatty fish. There are two types of fats: saturated and unsaturated. Saturated fats, such as those found in butter and red meat, should be consumed in moderation as they can increase cholesterol levels. Unsaturated fats, such as those found in avocados and olive oil, are considered healthy fats and should be consumed in larger amounts.

It is important to consume a balanced diet that includes all three macronutrients in the appropriate amounts. The exact amounts needed vary depending on factors such as age, gender, and activity level.

Recommended Ratio Of Macronutrients For Endomorphs

Endomorphs are individuals who tend to have a larger body frame and store fat easily. They may find it more difficult to lose weight and build muscle than individuals with other body types. However, with the right diet and exercise plan, endomorphs can achieve their fitness goals.

When it comes to macronutrients, endomorphs should focus on consuming a balanced diet with an appropriate ratio of carbohydrates, proteins, and fats. A common ratio for endomorphs is 40% carbohydrates, 30% protein, and 30% fat.

Carbohydrates are important for providing energy for workouts and other physical activity. However, endomorphs should focus on consuming complex carbohydrates, such as those found in whole grains and vegetables, rather than simple carbohydrates, such as those found in candy and sugary drinks. This will help prevent spikes in blood sugar levels and promote sustained energy.

Proteins are important for building and repairing muscle tissue. Endomorphs should aim to consume a variety of protein sources, including lean meats, poultry, fish, beans, and nuts. It is also important to consume protein throughout the day, rather than just at one meal, to promote muscle growth and repair.

Fats are important for hormone production and absorption of vitamins and minerals. Endomorphs should focus on consuming healthy fats, such as those found in avocados and olive oil, in moderation. It is also important to limit saturated fats, such as those found in butter and red meat.

It is important for endomorphs to consume a balanced diet with appropriate amounts of all three macronutrients. It may also be beneficial for them to work with a registered dietitian or nutritionist to develop a personalized plan that meets their individual needs and goals.

How The Endomorph Diet Supports Weight Loss And Muscle Building

The endomorph diet can be beneficial for both weight loss and muscle building. By consuming a balanced diet with an appropriate ratio of macronutrients, endomorphs can provide their bodies with the necessary nutrients to support their goals.

Weight loss can be achieved by consuming fewer calories than the body burns through physical activity and normal bodily functions. Endomorphs may find it more difficult to lose weight due to their tendency to store fat easily. However, by focusing on consuming complex carbohydrates, lean proteins, and healthy fats, endomorphs can promote sustained energy and avoid spikes in blood sugar levels. This can help prevent overeating and promote weight loss.

Muscle building requires a combination of resistance training and proper nutrition. Endomorphs may have an advantage when it comes to building muscle due to their larger body frame. However, it is still important to consume a balanced diet with an appropriate ratio of macronutrients. Consuming protein throughout the day can help promote muscle growth and repair, while carbohydrates provide energy for workouts.

In addition to proper nutrition, endomorphs should also focus on resistance training to build muscle. This can include exercises such as weightlifting, bodyweight exercises, and resistance band training. Consistency and progression are key when it comes to building muscle, so it is important to gradually increase the weight or resistance used during workouts.

Overall, the endomorph diet can support both weight loss and muscle building when combined with regular physical activity and a balanced diet. It is important for endomorphs to work with a registered dietitian or nutritionist to develop a personalized plan that meets their individual needs and goals.

CHAPTER THREE

FOODS TO EAT AND
FOODS TO AVOID

Foods Recommended For The Endomorph Diet

The endomorph body type tends to gain weight easily, and it can be challenging to shed that weight once it's been gained. However, the right diet can help endomorphs achieve their weight loss goals. Here are some of the foods that are recommended for the endomorph diet:

1. Protein

Protein is an essential nutrient for building and repairing muscle tissue. It's also beneficial for weight loss because it helps keep you feeling full for longer periods. Endomorphs should aim to consume a good amount of protein with each meal to keep their metabolism high and prevent muscle loss. Good sources of protein include lean meats, fish, eggs, legumes, and dairy products.

2. Vegetables

Vegetables are low in calories and high in nutrients, making them an excellent addition to any diet. Endomorphs should aim to consume a variety of vegetables, including leafy greens, broccoli, cauliflower, bell peppers, and mushrooms. Vegetables can help fill you up and provide essential vitamins and minerals to support weight loss.

3. Whole Grains

Whole grains are an excellent source of fiber, which can help endomorphs feel fuller for longer periods. They also provide essential vitamins and minerals, such as B vitamins and iron. Endomorphs should choose whole-grain options such as brown rice, quinoa, and whole-grain bread over refined grains like white rice and white bread.

4. Healthy Fats

Endomorphs should aim to consume healthy fats, such as those found in avocados, nuts, seeds, and fatty fish. Healthy fats can help improve satiety and boost metabolism, leading to weight loss.

5. Fruits

Fruits are an excellent source of vitamins, minerals, and fiber. Endomorphs should aim to consume a variety of fruits, including berries, apples, oranges, and bananas. However, they should be mindful of portion sizes and avoid consuming too much fruit, which can lead to weight gain.

Explanation Of Why These Foods Are Beneficial

The foods listed above are beneficial for endomorphs because they provide essential nutrients to support weight loss. Protein, for example, is essential for building and repairing muscle tissue, which can help improve metabolism and prevent muscle loss during weight loss. Vegetables and whole grains are low in calories and high in fiber, helping endomorphs feel fuller for longer periods and reducing the likelihood of overeating.

Healthy fats are also essential for endomorphs because

they can help improve satiety and boost metabolism. Fruits provide essential vitamins, minerals, and fiber, but endomorphs should be mindful of portion sizes to avoid consuming too many calories. By incorporating these foods into their diet, endomorphs can support their weight loss goals and improve overall health.

Foods To Avoid Or Limit On The Endomorph Diet

While some foods can help endomorphs achieve their weight loss goals, others can be detrimental. Here are some of the foods that endomorphs should avoid or limit on their diet:

1. Processed Foods

Processed foods are often high in calories, sugar, and unhealthy fats. They can also be low in nutrients, which can lead to overeating and weight gain. Endomorphs should limit their consumption of processed foods and opt for whole, nutrient-dense foods instead.

2. Sugary Drinks

Sugary drinks, such as soda and fruit juice, are high in sugar and calories, leading to weight gain. Endomorphs should avoid sugary drinks and opt for water, tea, or other low-calorie beverages.

3. Refined Carbohydrates

Refined carbohydrates, such as white bread, white rice, and pasta, are low in fiber and can cause a rapid increase in blood sugar levels, leading to insulin spikes and weight gain. Endomorphs should opt for whole-grain alternatives to refined carbohydrates.

4. Fried Foods

Fried foods are high in unhealthy fats, which can increase the risk of heart disease and weight gain. Endomorphs should avoid fried foods and opt for baked or grilled options instead.

5. High-Fat Meats

High-fat meats, such as bacon, sausage, and fatty cuts

of beef, can be high in calories and unhealthy fats. Endomorphs should opt for leaner cuts of meat, such as skinless chicken breast, fish, and lean beef.

Explanation Of Why These Foods Can Be Detrimental

The foods listed above can be detrimental to endomorphs because they can contribute to weight gain and negatively affect overall health. Processed foods are often high in calories, sugar, and unhealthy fats, which can lead to overeating and weight gain. Sugary drinks are also high in sugar and calories, leading to insulin spikes and weight gain.

Refined carbohydrates are low in fiber and can cause a rapid increase in blood sugar levels, leading to insulin spikes and weight gain. Fried foods are high in unhealthy fats, which can increase the risk of heart disease and weight gain. High-fat meats can also be high in calories and unhealthy fats, contributing to weight gain.

By avoiding or limiting these foods in their diet,

endomorphs can support their weight loss goals and improve overall health. Opting for whole, nutrient-dense foods and avoiding processed, high-calorie options can make a significant difference in achieving weight loss and maintaining a healthy body weight.

CHAPTER FOUR

EXERCISE AND THE ENDOMORPH DIET

Explanation Of The Role Of Exercise In Weight Loss And Muscle Building For Endomorphs

Endomorphs are individuals who tend to gain weight easily and struggle with losing weight. They have a slower metabolism, which makes it harder for them to burn calories compared to other body types. However, exercise can play a crucial role in helping endomorphs achieve their weight loss and muscle building goals.

One of the benefits of exercise for endomorphs is that it can increase their metabolic rate. By engaging in regular physical activity, endomorphs can boost their metabolism and burn more calories, even when at rest. This means that they can lose weight more easily and maintain a healthy weight in the long term.

Exercise also helps endomorphs build muscle, which is important for weight loss and overall health. Muscle tissue is more metabolically active than fat tissue, meaning that the more muscle an individual has, the more calories they burn at rest. By building muscle through exercise, endomorphs can increase their metabolic rate and burn more calories, even when not exercising.

In addition to weight loss and muscle building, exercise also offers numerous other health benefits for endomorphs. Regular physical activity can help lower blood pressure, reduce the risk of heart disease and stroke, improve bone density, and boost overall mood and mental health.

However, it's important to note that exercise alone is not enough for weight loss and muscle building for endomorphs. Diet also plays a crucial role in achieving these goals. Endomorphs should focus on a balanced diet that includes lean protein, healthy fats, complex carbohydrates, and plenty of fruits and vegetables. By combining exercise with a healthy diet, endomorphs can achieve their weight loss and muscle building goals more effectively.

Recommended Types Of Exercise For Endomorphs

While any type of exercise can benefit endomorphs, there are some types of exercise that may be more effective for weight loss and muscle building. Here are some recommended types of exercise for endomorphs:

Resistance Training

Resistance training, such as weightlifting, is an effective way for endomorphs to build muscle and increase their metabolic rate. By lifting weights or using resistance bands, endomorphs can target specific muscle groups and build lean muscle mass. This, in turn, helps them burn more calories at rest and achieve their weight loss and muscle building goals.

High-Intensity Interval Training (HIIT)

HIIT involves short bursts of intense exercise followed by periods of rest or low-intensity exercise. This type of exercise has been shown to be effective for weight loss and building cardiovascular endurance. Endomorphs can try HIIT workouts that incorporate bodyweight exercises, such as squats, lunges, and push-ups, for a full-body workout.

Cardiovascular Exercise

Cardiovascular exercise, such as running, swimming, or cycling, can also be effective for weight loss and improving cardiovascular health. Endomorphs should aim for at least 30 minutes of moderate-intensity cardiovascular exercise most days of the week.

Yoga and Pilates

Yoga and Pilates are low-impact exercises that focus on building strength, flexibility, and balance. These types of exercises can be beneficial for endomorphs who may have joint pain or mobility issues. They can also help improve posture and reduce stress levels.

Tips For Incorporating Exercise Into A Busy Lifestyle

For many endomorphs, incorporating regular exercise into a busy lifestyle can be a challenge. Here are some tips to help make exercise a habit:

Schedule Exercise Time

Endomorphs should treat exercise like any other appointment and schedule it into their day. This can help them make it a priority and ensure that they have time for it in their busy schedule.

Find an Exercise Buddy

Working out with a friend or family member can make exercise more enjoyable and help hold endomorphs accountable. They can motivate each other to stick to their fitness goals and make exercise a social activity.

Choose Activities You Enjoy

Endomorphs should choose activities they enjoy, as this can help make exercise feel less like a chore. They can try different types of exercise until they find something they truly enjoy, whether it's hiking, dancing, or playing a sport.

Make Exercise a Part of Daily Routine

Endomorphs can incorporate exercise into their daily routine by taking the stairs instead of the elevator, walking or biking to work, or taking a lunchtime walk. These small changes can add up over time and help them stay active even on busy days.

Try Short Workouts

Endomorphs can try short workouts, such as 10-minute sessions of high-intensity interval training, throughout the day if they don't have time for a longer workout. This can help them stay active and break up long periods of sitting.

Be Flexible

Finally, endomorphs should be flexible with their exercise routine and not be too hard on themselves if they miss a workout. They should focus on making exercise a habit and finding ways to fit it into their busy lifestyle, rather than striving for perfection.

In conclusion, exercise can play a crucial role in weight loss and muscle building for endomorphs. By incorporating resistance training, high-intensity interval training, cardiovascular exercise, and yoga or Pilates into their routine, endomorphs can build lean muscle mass, boost their metabolism, and improve overall health. By scheduling exercise time, finding an exercise buddy, choosing activities they enjoy, making exercise a part of their daily routine, and being flexible, endomorphs can make exercise a habit and achieve their fitness goals.

Explanation Of The Role Of Exercise In Weight Loss And Muscle Building For Endomorphs

Endomorphs are individuals who tend to store more fat and have a slower metabolism. This can make it more difficult for them to lose weight and build muscle compared to other body types. However, exercise can play a crucial role in helping endomorphs achieve their weight loss and muscle building goals.

Weight Loss

Endomorphs who are looking to lose weight should focus on a combination of cardiovascular exercise and resistance training. Cardiovascular exercise, such as running, cycling, or swimming, can help endomorphs burn calories and improve their cardiovascular health. Resistance training, such as weightlifting or bodyweight exercises, can help endomorphs build lean muscle mass and boost their metabolism.

Studies have shown that high-intensity interval training (HIIT) can be particularly effective for weight loss in endomorphs. HIIT involves short bursts of intense exercise followed by periods of rest or low-intensity exercise. This type of training can help endomorphs burn more calories in a shorter amount of time compared to traditional steady-state cardio.

Muscle Building

Endomorphs who are looking to build muscle should focus on resistance training, with a particular emphasis on heavy lifting. Heavy lifting can help endomorphs build muscle and increase their strength. In addition, incorporating compound exercises, which work multiple muscle groups at once, can be particularly effective for building muscle.

Endomorphs should also pay attention to their diet when it comes to building muscle. Eating a diet rich in protein can help support muscle growth and repair. Aim for around 1 gram of protein per pound of body weight per day.

In addition to resistance training, endomorphs may also benefit from incorporating yoga or Pilates into their routine. These types of exercises can help improve flexibility, balance, and core strength, which can be particularly important for endomorphs who may have difficulty with certain exercises due to their body type.

In conclusion, exercise can play a crucial role in weight loss and muscle building for endomorphs. By incorporating a combination of cardiovascular exercise and resistance training, endomorphs can burn calories, build lean muscle mass, and boost their metabolism. In addition, heavy lifting, compound exercises, and a diet rich in protein can be particularly effective for building muscle. Yoga or Pilates can also be beneficial for improving flexibility, balance, and core strength.

Overcoming Challenges And Staying Motivated

Common Challenges Faced by Endomorphs when Following the Diet and Exercise Plan

Following a diet and exercise plan can be challenging for anyone, but endomorphs may face particular obstacles due to their body type. Some of the common challenges faced by endomorphs when following a diet and exercise plan include:

Difficulty Losing Weight

Endomorphs may struggle to lose weight due to their slower metabolism and tendency to store more fat. This can be frustrating and may make it harder to stick to a diet and exercise plan.

Fatigue and Low Energy

Endomorphs may also struggle with fatigue and low energy, which can make it harder to stick to an exercise routine.

Difficulty with Certain Exercises

Due to their body type, endomorphs may have difficulty with certain exercises, such as running or high-impact activities.

Cravings and Hunger

Endomorphs may also struggle with cravings and hunger, which can make it harder to stick to a healthy diet.

Strategies for Overcoming these Challenges

While these challenges can be difficult to overcome, there are strategies that can help endomorphs stick to their diet and exercise plan:

Focus on Small Changes

Rather than trying to make drastic changes to your diet

and exercise routine, focus on making small, sustainable changes. This could include adding more vegetables to your meals, taking a walk after dinner, or doing a short workout in the morning.

Prioritize Sleep and Recovery

Endomorphs may need more rest and recovery time than other body types. Prioritizing sleep and rest can help improve energy levels and reduce fatigue.

Find Exercise that Works for You

Endomorphs may have difficulty with certain exercises, but that doesn't mean they should give up on exercise altogether. Instead, focus on finding exercises that work for your body type, such as swimming or weightlifting.

Plan Ahead for Cravings and Hunger

To avoid giving in to cravings and hunger, plan ahead by packing healthy snacks or having a nutritious meal ready to go when hunger strikes.

Tips for Staying Motivated and on Track

Sticking to a diet and exercise plan can be challenging, but there are strategies that can help endomorphs stay motivated and on track:

Set Realistic Goals

Setting realistic goals can help keep you motivated and on track. Instead of aiming to lose 10 pounds in a week, set a goal to lose 1-2 pounds per week.

Find a Support System

Having a support system can help keep you accountable and motivated. This could include a workout buddy, a nutritionist, or a support group.

Track Your Progress

Tracking your progress can help you see how far you've come and keep you motivated to continue. This could include taking progress photos, keeping a food diary, or tracking your workouts.

Celebrate Your Successes

Don't forget to celebrate your successes along the way, no matter how small they may be. Reward yourself for sticking to your diet and exercise plan with a massage, a new workout outfit, or a night out with friends.

In conclusion, while endomorphs may face particular challenges when it comes to following a diet and exercise plan, there are strategies that can help them overcome these obstacles. By focusing on small changes, prioritizing sleep and recovery, finding exercise that works for your body type, and planning ahead for cravings and hunger, endomorphs can stick to their diet and exercise plan and achieve their health and fitness goals. Staying motivated and on track can also be achieved by setting realistic goals, finding a support system, tracking progress, and celebrating successes.

Supplementation For Endomorphs

Explanation of the Role of Supplements in the Endomorph Diet

Endomorphs are individuals with a body type characterized by a larger bone structure, higher body fat percentage, and a slower metabolism. This body type tends to gain weight quickly and have difficulty losing it. The Endomorph diet focuses on a low-carbohydrate, high-protein, and high-fat approach to help manage weight and improve health. Supplements can play a significant role in supporting this diet by providing essential nutrients that may be lacking in the diet or optimizing specific functions in the body.

Supplements can provide a variety of benefits for endomorphs, including supporting weight management, reducing inflammation, improving energy levels, and enhancing muscle growth. The Endomorph diet typically focuses on whole foods and limits processed foods and refined carbohydrates, which can lead to nutrient deficiencies. Supplements can help fill these nutrient gaps, ensuring optimal health and performance.

Supplements can also support weight management by boosting metabolism, reducing appetite, and improving insulin sensitivity. For example, caffeine and green tea extract are commonly used to increase metabolism and fat burning. Fiber supplements, such as psyllium husk, can help reduce appetite and improve digestive health, leading to more significant weight loss.

In addition to weight management, supplements can also improve overall health and well-being. Omega-3 fatty acids, found in fish oil supplements, can reduce inflammation and improve heart health. Vitamin D supplements can improve immune function and bone health. Probiotics can enhance gut health, which plays a critical role in overall health and weight management.

However, it is essential to remember that supplements should not replace a healthy diet. They are meant to supplement and optimize the diet, not to be the sole source of nutrition. It is also crucial to speak with a healthcare provider before starting any new supplements to ensure they are safe and appropriate for individual needs and health conditions.

Recommended Supplements for Endomorphs

Several supplements can benefit endomorphs by supporting weight management, improving health, and enhancing performance. Here are some recommended supplements for endomorphs:

1. Protein Supplements - Protein supplements can help endomorphs reach their daily protein intake requirements and support muscle growth and repair. Whey protein is a popular option as it is quickly absorbed and contains all essential amino acids.

2. Omega-3 Fatty Acids - Omega-3 fatty acids can reduce inflammation and improve heart health, which is particularly important for endomorphs who may be at higher risk of heart disease. Fish oil supplements are a good source of omega-3s.

3. Fiber Supplements - Fiber supplements can help reduce appetite, improve digestion, and support weight management. Psyllium husk is a common option.

4. Probiotics - Probiotics can enhance gut health, which is essential for overall health and weight management. Look for a high-quality probiotic supplement with a variety of strains.

5. Vitamin D - Many endomorphs are deficient

in vitamin D, which can lead to several health problems, including weakened immune function and bone health. A vitamin D supplement can help ensure adequate intake.

6. Caffeine - Caffeine can increase metabolism and fat burning, making it a popular supplement for weight management. However, it is essential to use caffeine supplements in moderation and be aware of potential side effects.

Benefits And Risks Of Supplementation

While supplements can provide several benefits for endomorphs, there are also potential risks to be aware of. One risk is the potential for nutrient toxicity if taking high doses of certain vitamins and minerals. For example, taking too much vitamin A can lead to liver damage, while excessive iron intake can cause digestive issues and liver damage.

Another risk is the potential for interactions with medications. Some supplements can interact with prescription medications, leading to adverse effects or reducing the effectiveness of the medication. It is crucial to speak with a healthcare provider before starting any new supplements to ensure they are safe and appropriate for individual needs and health conditions.

There is also the risk of using supplements as a replacement for a healthy diet. While supplements can provide additional nutrients, they should not be relied upon as the sole source of nutrition. It is crucial to maintain a balanced and nutritious diet while using supplements to optimize health and performance.

However, when used appropriately and with guidance from a healthcare provider, supplements can provide several benefits for endomorphs. They can help support weight management, improve overall health, and enhance performance. It is essential to choose high-quality supplements from reputable brands and to follow dosing guidelines carefully to minimize risks and maximize benefits.

Eating Out And Traveling On The Endomorph Diet

Tips for Making Healthy Food Choices When Eating Out

Eating out can be a challenge when you are trying to maintain a healthy diet. Many restaurant meals are high in calories, fat, and sodium, and it can be difficult to know what to choose. However, with a little planning and some smart choices, you can enjoy a healthy meal out without sabotaging your diet. Here are some tips for making healthy food choices when eating out:

1. Plan ahead

Before you head out to the restaurant, take a look at the menu online. Most restaurants have their menus posted on their websites, and this can give you an idea of what options are available. Look for dishes that are grilled, roasted, or steamed, and avoid anything that is fried or comes with a creamy sauce.

2. Watch portion sizes

Many restaurants serve oversized portions, so be mindful of how much you are eating. Consider splitting a meal with a friend or taking half of it home for later.

3. Choose lean protein

When choosing a main dish, opt for lean protein sources such as grilled chicken or fish, instead of red meat or pork. Vegetarian options such as tofu or beans can also be a good choice.

4. Load up on veggies

Vegetables are a great way to fill up without consuming too many calories. Look for dishes that feature vegetables as the main ingredient or ask for extra veggies on the side.

5. Be mindful of condiments

Condiments such as dressings, sauces, and dips can be high in calories and fat. Ask for them on the side and use them sparingly.

6. Limit alcohol

Alcohol is high in calories and can lead to poor food choices. Limit your intake or choose a low-calorie option such as wine or light beer.

7. Don't be afraid to ask questions

If you are unsure about how a dish is prepared or what ingredients are used, don't be afraid to ask your server. Most restaurants are happy to accommodate dietary restrictions or preferences.

By following these tips, you can make healthy food choices when eating out and still enjoy your meal. Remember, moderation is key, and it's okay to indulge once in a while.

Strategies for Staying on Track While Traveling

Traveling can be a great way to experience new cultures and cuisines, but it can also be a challenge when you are trying to stay on track with your healthy habits. Being away from home can make it difficult to stick to a routine, and the temptation to indulge in unhealthy foods and skip workouts can be strong. However, with a little planning and some smart strategies, you can stay on track with your healthy habits while traveling. Here are some strategies for staying on track while traveling:

1. Pack healthy snacks

Bring along healthy snacks such as nuts, fruit, and protein bars to help you resist the temptation of unhealthy options while on the road or at the airport. This can also help you avoid going too long without eating, which can lead to poor food choices later on.

2. Stay hydrated

Traveling can be dehydrating, so be sure to drink plenty of water throughout the day. This can help you feel more energized and alert, and can also help you resist the temptation to overeat.

3. Plan ahead

Research healthy restaurants or grocery stores in the area where you will be staying. This can help you plan meals in advance and avoid the temptation of unhealthy options.

4. Stick to your routine

Try to stick to your regular routine as much as possible. This can include waking up at the same time each day, exercising at the same time, and sticking to regular meal times. This can help you maintain a sense of normalcy and prevent overindulging.

CHAPTER FIVE

MEAL PLANNING AND PREPARATION

Tips For Meal Planning On The Endomorph Diet

The endomorph diet is a nutrition plan that is tailored towards individuals with an endomorphic body type. Endomorphs are individuals who have a slower metabolism, which means they are more prone to gaining weight and storing fat. To combat this, meal planning is a crucial component of the endomorph diet. Here are some tips to help with meal planning on the endomorph diet:

1. Focus on Whole Foods

One of the most important aspects of the endomorph diet is consuming whole, nutrient-dense foods. Whole foods are foods that are minimally processed and do not contain added sugars, artificial preservatives, or other additives. Examples of whole foods include fruits, vegetables, whole grains, lean proteins, and healthy fats.

2. Watch Your Carbohydrate Intake

While carbohydrates are an essential macronutrient, consuming too many can be detrimental to endomorphs as their bodies are less efficient at metabolizing them. When planning meals, endomorphs should aim to consume complex carbohydrates such as whole grains, vegetables, and fruits rather than refined carbohydrates such as white bread, sugary drinks, and desserts.

3. Don't Skip Meals

Skipping meals can cause blood sugar levels to fluctuate, leading to cravings and overeating. Endomorphs should aim to eat small, frequent meals throughout the day to keep their blood sugar levels stable and prevent overeating.

4. Incorporate Protein with Every Meal

Protein is essential for building and repairing muscle tissue, and it also helps keep endomorphs feeling full and satisfied. When planning meals, endomorphs should aim to incorporate a source of lean protein with every meal, such as chicken, fish, tofu, or beans.

5. Practice Portion Control

Endomorphs are more prone to overeating and weight gain, so practicing portion control is crucial. Using smaller plates and measuring food portions can help with portion control and prevent overeating.

Sample Meal Plans For A Week

Here are some sample meal plans for a week that are suitable for endomorphs:

Monday

- Breakfast: Oatmeal with berries and almonds
- Snack: Greek yogurt with fruit
- Lunch: Grilled chicken salad with mixed greens, tomatoes, and avocado
- Snack: Apple slices with almond butter
- Dinner: Baked salmon with roasted vegetables

Tuesday

- Breakfast: Scrambled eggs with spinach and

whole grain toast

- Snack: Carrots and hummus
- Lunch: Quinoa bowl with grilled chicken, mixed vegetables, and avocado
- Snack: Cottage cheese with fruit
- Dinner: Turkey meatballs with zucchini noodles and marinara sauce

Wednesday

- Breakfast: Greek yogurt with granola and berries
- Snack: Apple slices with peanut butter
- Lunch: Lentil soup with mixed greens and a whole grain roll
- Snack: Celery sticks with hummus
- Dinner: Grilled flank steak with roasted sweet potatoes and asparagus

Thursday

- Breakfast: Smoothie with Greek yogurt, berries, and spinach
- Snack: Hard-boiled eggs
- Lunch: Chicken wrap with mixed greens, avocado, and whole grain wrap
- Snack: Almonds and dried fruit
- Dinner: Stir-fry with tofu, mixed vegetables, and brown rice

Friday

- Breakfast: Breakfast burrito with scrambled eggs, black beans, and salsa

- Snack: Baby carrots and hummus

- Lunch: Grilled chicken Caesar salad with whole grain croutons

- Snack: Greek yogurt with honey

- Dinner: Baked cod with roasted vegetables and quinoa

Saturday

- Breakfast: Whole grain waffles with almond butter and banana slices

- Snack: Greek yogurt with granola

- Lunch: Grilled chicken sandwich with mixed greens and whole grain bread

- Snack: Fresh fruit salad

- Dinner: Grilled shrimp skewers with mixed vegetables and quinoa

Sunday

- Breakfast: Scrambled eggs with whole grain toast and sliced avocado

- Snack: Apple slices with almond butter

- Lunch: Tuna salad with mixed greens and whole grain crackers

- Snack: Mixed nuts

- Dinner: Baked chicken with roasted vegetables and brown rice

It's important to note that these meal plans are just examples, and endomorphs should adjust their meals to fit their individual needs and preferences.

CHAPTER SIX

RECIPE IDEAS FOR ENDOMORPH-FRIENDLY MEALS AND SNACKS

Grilled Chicken Breast with Roasted Sweet Potatoes and Steamed Broccoli

Description

This meal is a healthy and flavorful option that is perfect for lunch or dinner. Grilled chicken breast is paired with roasted sweet potatoes and steamed broccoli for a well-rounded and satisfying meal.

Ingredients

- 4 boneless, skinless chicken breasts
- 2 medium sweet potatoes, peeled and cut into 1-inch pieces
- 1 head of broccoli, cut into florets
- 2 tablespoons olive oil
- 1 teaspoon garlic powder
- 1 teaspoon paprika
- Salt and pepper to taste

Instructions

1. Preheat the oven to 425°F.

2. In a large bowl, toss the sweet potatoes with 1 tablespoon of olive oil, garlic powder, paprika, salt, and pepper.

3. Arrange the sweet potatoes in a single layer on a baking sheet and roast for 20-25 minutes or until tender and lightly browned.

4. Season the chicken breasts with salt and pepper to taste.

5. Heat a grill pan over medium-high heat and brush with 1 tablespoon of olive oil.

6. Grill the chicken breasts for 6-8 minutes per side or until cooked through.

7. While the chicken and sweet potatoes are cooking, steam the broccoli for 3-4 minutes or until tender.

8. Serve the grilled chicken with roasted sweet potatoes and steamed broccoli.

Nutritional Information

- Calories: 360
- Protein: 38g
- Carbohydrates: 27g
- Fat: 10g

- Fiber: 6g

Turkey Meatballs with Zucchini Noodles and Tomato Sauce

Description

This meal is a healthy and delicious option that is perfect for a low-carb dinner. Turkey meatballs are served with zucchini noodles and a flavorful tomato sauce for a satisfying and nutritious meal.

Ingredients

For the Meatballs:

- 1 pound ground turkey
- 1 egg
- 1/2 cup almond flour
- 1/4 cup chopped fresh parsley
- 1/4 cup chopped fresh basil
- 1 teaspoon garlic powder
- Salt and pepper to taste

For the Sauce:

- 1 tablespoon olive oil

- 1 small onion, diced
- 2 garlic cloves, minced
- 1 can (14.5 oz) diced tomatoes
- 1/4 teaspoon red pepper flakes
- Salt and pepper to taste

For the Zucchini Noodles:

- 2 medium zucchini, spiralized
- Salt and pepper to taste

Instructions

1. Preheat the oven to 400°F.

2. In a large bowl, mix together the ground turkey, egg, almond flour, parsley, basil, garlic powder, salt, and pepper until well combined.

3. Form the mixture into meatballs, about 2 tablespoons each, and place them on a baking sheet lined with parchment paper.

4. Bake for 20-25 minutes or until the meatballs are cooked through and lightly browned.

5. While the meatballs are cooking, make the tomato sauce. Heat the olive oil in a large skillet over medium heat.

6. Add the onion and garlic and sauté until softened, about 5 minutes.

7. Add the diced tomatoes, red pepper flakes, salt, and pepper and simmer for 10-15 minutes or until the sauce has thickened.

8. While the sauce is simmering, spiralize the zucchini into noodles and sprinkle with salt and pepper to taste.

9. When the meatballs are done, serve them with the zucchini noodles and tomato sauce.

Baked Salmon with Quinoa and Roasted Asparagus

Description

This meal is packed with healthy omega-3 fatty acids and is a great option for a nutritious dinner. Baked salmon is served with quinoa and roasted asparagus for a well-balanced and flavorful meal.

Ingredients

- 4 salmon fillets (6 oz each)
- 1 cup quinoa, rinsed and drained
- 2 cups water
- 1 bunch asparagus, tough ends trimmed
- 2 tablespoons olive oil
- Salt and pepper to taste

- Lemon wedges for serving

Instructions

1. Preheat the oven to 400°F.

2. In a medium saucepan, bring the water to a boil over high heat. Add the quinoa and reduce the heat to low. Cover and simmer for 15-20 minutes or until the quinoa is tender and the water has been absorbed.

3. Arrange the asparagus on a baking sheet and drizzle with 1 tablespoon of olive oil. Season with salt and pepper to taste.

4. Roast for 10-12 minutes or until tender and lightly browned.

5. Season the salmon fillets with salt and pepper to taste.

6. Heat a large oven-safe skillet over medium-high heat and add the remaining 1 tablespoon of olive oil.

7. Add the salmon fillets to the skillet and cook for 2-3 minutes per side or until lightly browned.

8. Transfer the skillet to the oven and bake for 10-12 minutes or until the salmon is cooked through.

9. Serve the salmon with quinoa and roasted asparagus. Squeeze lemon wedges over the top, if desired.

Nutritional Information

- Calories: 450
- Protein: 38g
- Carbohydrates: 30g
- Fat: 19g
- Fiber: 5g

Ground Turkey Chili with Kidney Beans and Bell Peppers

Description

This hearty and flavorful chili is a great option for a cozy dinner. Ground turkey is simmered with kidney beans and bell peppers in a rich and savory tomato-based sauce for a comforting and satisfying meal.

Ingredients

- 1 pound ground turkey
- 1 onion, chopped
- 1 green bell pepper, chopped
- 1 red bell pepper, chopped
- 2 garlic cloves, minced

- 1 can (14.5 oz) diced tomatoes

- 1 can (15 oz) kidney beans, drained and rinsed

- 1 tablespoon chili powder

- 1 teaspoon cumin

- Salt and pepper to taste

- Optional toppings: shredded cheese, sour cream, chopped cilantro

Instructions

1. Heat a large pot over medium-high heat.

2. Add the ground turkey and cook, breaking it up with a wooden spoon, until browned and cooked through, about 8-10 minutes.

3. Add the onion, bell peppers, and garlic and sauté until softened, about 5 minutes.

4. Add the diced tomatoes, kidney beans, chili powder, cumin, salt, and pepper and stir to combine.

5. Bring the mixture to a simmer and reduce the heat to low.

6. Cover and simmer for 20-30 minutes or until the chili has thickened and the flavors have melded together.

7. Serve hot with your choice of toppings, if desired.

Nutritional Information

- Calories: 350
- Protein: 29g
- Carbohydrates: 35g
- Fat: 11g
- Fiber: 9g

Grilled Steak with Roasted Root Vegetables and Sautéed Spinach

Description

This meal is a classic combination of a juicy grilled steak with roasted root vegetables and sautéed spinach. It's a satisfying and nutritious dinner that's sure to please.

Ingredients

- 1 pound sirloin steak
- 2 medium sweet potatoes, peeled and cut into 1-inch cubes
- 2 medium carrots, peeled and cut into 1-inch pieces
- 2 parsnips, peeled and cut into 1-inch pieces
- 2 tablespoons olive oil

- Salt and pepper to taste

- 1 tablespoon butter

- 2 garlic cloves, minced

- 6 cups fresh spinach leaves

Instructions

1. Preheat the grill to medium-high heat.

2. Season the steak with salt and pepper to taste.

3. Grill the steak for 4-6 minutes per side or until desired doneness is reached.

4. Remove the steak from the grill and let it rest for 5 minutes before slicing.

5. Meanwhile, preheat the oven to 400°F.

6. Place the sweet potatoes, carrots, and parsnips on a baking sheet and toss with olive oil. Season with salt and pepper to taste.

7. Roast for 25-30 minutes or until the vegetables are tender and lightly browned.

8. Melt the butter in a large skillet over medium heat.

9. Add the garlic and sauté for 1-2 minutes or until fragrant.

10. Add the spinach and sauté for 2-3 minutes or until wilted.

11. Serve the sliced steak with roasted root

vegetables and sautéed spinach.

Nutritional Information

- Calories: 450
- Protein: 32g
- Carbohydrates: 27g
- Fat: 24g
- Fiber: 6g

Black Bean and Vegetable Stir-Fry with Brown Rice

Description

This vegetarian stir-fry is loaded with protein and fiber from black beans and vegetables. Served with brown rice, it's a delicious and nutritious meal that's quick and easy to make.

Ingredients

- 2 cups cooked brown rice
- 1 tablespoon vegetable oil
- 1 onion, sliced
- 1 red bell pepper, sliced

- 1 green bell pepper, sliced
- 1 zucchini, sliced
- 1 can (15 oz) black beans, drained and rinsed
- 2 garlic cloves, minced
- 2 teaspoons ground cumin
- Salt and pepper to taste

Instructions

1. Heat the vegetable oil in a large skillet or wok over high heat.

2. Add the onion, bell peppers, and zucchini and stir-fry for 3-4 minutes or until the vegetables are tender-crisp.

3. Add the black beans, garlic, cumin, salt, and pepper and stir-fry for 1-2 minutes or until heated through.

4. Serve the stir-fry over cooked brown rice.

Nutritional Information

- Calories: 400
- Protein: 13g
- Carbohydrates: 70g
- Fat: 7g
- Fiber: 13g

Spicy Turkey and Vegetable Soup

Description

This soup is a delicious and comforting meal that's perfect for cold days. Made with ground turkey and vegetables, it's a healthy and filling option that's also easy to make.

Ingredients

- 1 pound ground turkey
- 1 onion, chopped
- 2 garlic cloves, minced
- 1 red bell pepper, chopped
- 1 green bell pepper, chopped
- 2 cups sliced carrots
- 1 can (15 oz) diced tomatoes
- 6 cups chicken or vegetable broth
- 1 teaspoon paprika
- 1/2 teaspoon cumin
- 1/2 teaspoon chili powder
- Salt and pepper to taste
- 2 tablespoons chopped fresh cilantro

Instructions

1. Heat a large pot over medium-high heat.

2. Add the ground turkey and cook, breaking it up with a spoon, until browned.

3. Add the onion, garlic, red and green bell peppers, and carrots and sauté for 5-7 minutes or until the vegetables are tender.

4. Add the diced tomatoes, broth, paprika, cumin, chili powder, salt, and pepper and stir to combine.

5. Bring the soup to a boil, then reduce the heat and simmer for 20-30 minutes or until the vegetables are tender and the flavors have blended.

6. Stir in the chopped cilantro and serve hot.

Nutritional Information

- Calories: 250
- Protein: 21g
- Carbohydrates: 19g
- Fat: 9g
- Fiber: 5g

Grilled Shrimp Skewers with Mixed Grilled Vegetables

Description

These grilled shrimp skewers are a delicious and healthy meal that's perfect for summer. Paired with mixed grilled vegetables, they're a flavorful and nutritious option for any day of the week.

Ingredients

- 1 pound large shrimp, peeled and deveined
- 2 tablespoons olive oil
- 1 tablespoon fresh lemon juice
- 1 tablespoon chopped fresh parsley
- Salt and pepper to taste
- 1 red bell pepper, seeded and cut into 1-inch pieces
- 1 yellow bell pepper, seeded and cut into 1-inch pieces
- 1 zucchini, sliced
- 1 red onion, cut into wedges
- 8-10 wooden skewers, soaked in water for 30 minutes

Instructions

1. Preheat the grill to medium-high heat.

2. In a large bowl, whisk together the olive oil, lemon juice, parsley, salt, and pepper.

3. Add the shrimp to the bowl and toss to coat.

4. Thread the shrimp onto the skewers, alternating with the bell peppers, zucchini, and red onion.

5. Grill the skewers for 2-3 minutes per side or until the shrimp are cooked through and the vegetables are tender.

6. Serve the skewers with additional chopped parsley, if desired.

Nutritional Information

- Calories: 200
- Protein: 20g
- Carbohydrates: 10g
- Fat: 8g
- Fiber: 3g

Stuffed Bell Peppers with Ground Beef and Quinoa

Description

These stuffed bell peppers are a hearty and flavorful meal

that's perfect for a family dinner or meal prep. Made with ground beef and quinoa, they're packed with protein and nutrients.

Ingredients

- 4 bell peppers, tops cut off and seeds removed
- 1 pound lean ground beef
- 1 onion, chopped
- 2 garlic cloves, minced
- 1 cup cooked quinoa
- 1 can (15 oz) diced tomatoes
- 1 teaspoon paprika
- 1/2 teaspoon cumin
- Salt and pepper to taste
- 1/2 cup shredded cheddar cheese

Instructions

1. Preheat the oven to 375°F (190°C).

2. In a large skillet, cook the ground beef over medium-high heat until browned.

3. Add the onion and garlic to the skillet and sauté for 2-3 minutes or until softened.

4. Add the cooked quinoa, diced tomatoes,

paprika, cumin, salt, and pepper to the skillet and stir to combine.

5. Spoon the beef and quinoa mixture into each bell pepper.

6. Place the stuffed bell peppers in a baking dish and bake for 25-30 minutes or until the peppers are tender and the filling is hot.

7. Sprinkle the shredded cheddar cheese over the stuffed peppers and return to the oven for an additional 5 minutes or until the cheese is melted and bubbly.

Nutritional Information

- Calories: 350

- Protein: 30g

- Carbohydrates: 22g

- Fat: 16g

- Fiber: 6g

Chicken and Vegetable Curry with Brown Rice

Description

This chicken and vegetable curry is a flavorful and healthy meal that's easy to make. With a creamy coconut milk sauce and a variety of vegetables, it's a satisfying option for any day of the week.

Ingredients

- 1 pound boneless, skinless chicken breasts, cut into bite-sized pieces
- 1 onion, chopped
- 2 garlic cloves, minced
- 1 red bell pepper, seeded and chopped
- 1 green bell pepper, seeded and chopped
- 2 cups chopped mixed vegetables (such as zucchini, carrots, and mushrooms)
- 1 can (14 oz) coconut milk
- 1 tablespoon curry powder
- 1/2 teaspoon cumin
- Salt and pepper to taste
- 2 cups cooked brown rice

Instructions

1. In a large skillet, cook the chicken over medium-high heat until browned.

2. Add the onion, garlic, and bell peppers to the skillet and sauté for 2-3 minutes or until softened.

3. Add the mixed vegetables to the skillet and sauté for an additional 5-7 minutes or until

tender.

4. Stir in the coconut milk, curry powder, cumin, salt, and pepper and bring to a simmer.

5. Reduce the heat and simmer the curry for 15-20 minutes or until the chicken is cooked through and the sauce has thickened.

6. Serve the curry over cooked brown rice.

Nutritional Information

- Calories: 400
- Protein: 30g
- Carbohydrates: 30g
- Fat: 16g
- Fiber: 6g

Tuna Salad with Mixed Greens and Avocado

Description

This tuna salad is a refreshing and healthy meal that's perfect for lunch or dinner. Made with mixed greens, avocado, and a tangy lemon dressing, it's a satisfying option for anyone who loves seafood.

Ingredients

- 2 cans (5 oz each) tuna, drained
- 4 cups mixed greens
- 1 avocado, diced
- 1/4 red onion, sliced
- 1/4 cup chopped fresh parsley
- 1 lemon, juiced
- 2 tablespoons olive oil
- Salt and pepper to taste

Instructions

1. In a large bowl, combine the drained tuna, mixed greens, diced avocado, sliced red onion, and chopped parsley.

2. In a small bowl, whisk together the lemon juice, olive oil, salt, and pepper.

3. Pour the dressing over the salad and toss to combine.

4. Serve the tuna salad immediately.

Nutritional Information

- Calories: 350
- Protein: 30g
- Carbohydrates: 15g
- Fat: 20g

- Fiber: 8g

Roasted Pork Tenderloin with Roasted Brussels Sprouts and Sweet Potato Mash

Description

This roasted pork tenderloin is a delicious and satisfying meal that's perfect for a special occasion or a family dinner. Served with roasted Brussels sprouts and sweet potato mash, it's a complete and balanced meal.

Ingredients

- 1 pound pork tenderloin
- 1 tablespoon olive oil
- 1 teaspoon dried thyme
- Salt and pepper to taste
- 1 pound Brussels sprouts, trimmed and halved
- 2 sweet potatoes, peeled and diced
- 1/4 cup milk
- 1 tablespoon butter

Instructions

1. Preheat the oven to 400°F (200°C).

2. Rub the pork tenderloin with the olive oil, dried thyme, salt, and pepper.

3. Place the pork tenderloin on a baking sheet and roast for 25-30 minutes or until the internal temperature reaches 145°F (63°C).

4. While the pork tenderloin is roasting, toss the Brussels sprouts with olive oil, salt, and pepper.

5. Place the Brussels sprouts on a separate baking sheet and roast for 20-25 minutes or until tender and crispy.

6. In a large pot, cover the diced sweet potatoes with water and bring to a boil.

7. Reduce the heat and simmer the sweet potatoes for 10-15 minutes or until tender.

8. Drain the sweet potatoes and mash them with the milk and butter.

9. Slice the pork tenderloin and serve with the roasted Brussels sprouts and sweet potato mash.

Nutritional Information

- Calories: 400

- Protein: 30g

- Carbohydrates: 30g

- Fat: 16g

- Fiber: 8g

Lentil Soup with Mixed Vegetables

Description

This lentil soup is a hearty and flavorful meal that's perfect for a chilly day. Loaded with mixed vegetables and protein-packed lentils, it's a satisfying option for anyone who wants a healthy and comforting meal.

Ingredients

- 1 tablespoon olive oil
- 1 onion, chopped
- 2 garlic cloves, minced
- 2 carrots, chopped
- 2 celery stalks, chopped
- 1 teaspoon dried thyme
- 1 teaspoon smoked paprika
- 1/2 teaspoon cumin
- 1 cup lentils, rinsed and drained
- 4 cups vegetable broth
- 2 cups mixed vegetables (such as zucchini, green beans, and corn)
- Salt and pepper to taste

Instructions

1. In a large pot, heat the olive oil over medium heat.

2. Add the chopped onion and minced garlic and sauté for 3-5 minutes or until fragrant.

3. Add the chopped carrots, celery, dried thyme, smoked paprika, and cumin and sauté for another 5-7 minutes or until the vegetables are tender.

4. Add the rinsed and drained lentils and vegetable broth to the pot and bring to a boil.

5. Reduce the heat and simmer the soup for 30-35 minutes or until the lentils are tender.

6. Add the mixed vegetables and continue to simmer for another 10-15 minutes or until the vegetables are tender.

7. Season the soup with salt and pepper to taste.

8. Serve the lentil soup hot with crusty bread.

Nutritional Information

- Calories: 300
- Protein: 16g
- Carbohydrates: 46g
- Fat: 5g

- Fiber: 16g

Grilled Chicken Kabobs with Grilled Eggplant and Mixed Greens Salad

Description

These grilled chicken kabobs are a delicious and healthy meal that's perfect for a summer barbecue or a family dinner. Served with grilled eggplant and a mixed greens salad, they're a complete and balanced meal.

Ingredients

- 1 pound boneless, skinless chicken breasts, cut into cubes
- 1 eggplant, sliced
- 2 tablespoons olive oil
- 2 tablespoons balsamic vinegar
- 1 tablespoon Dijon mustard
- 1 garlic clove, minced
- Salt and pepper to taste
- 4 cups mixed greens
- 1/2 cup cherry tomatoes, halved
- 1/4 red onion, sliced
- 1/4 cup crumbled feta cheese

- 1/4 cup chopped fresh parsley

- 1 lemon, juiced

- 2 tablespoons olive oil

Instructions

1. Preheat the grill to medium-high heat.

2. Thread the chicken cubes onto skewers and brush with olive oil.

3. Brush the eggplant slices with olive oil and season with salt and pepper.

4. In a small bowl, whisk together the balsamic vinegar, Dijon mustard, minced garlic, salt, and pepper.

5. Grill the chicken kabobs and eggplant slices for 10-12 minutes or until cooked through.

6. In a large bowl, combine the mixed greens, cherry tomatoes, sliced red onion, crumbled feta cheese, and chopped fresh parsley.

7. In a small bowl, whisk together the lemon juice, olive oil, salt, and pepper.

8. Toss the mixed greens salad with the lemon dressing.

9. Serve the grilled chicken kabobs and eggplant slices with the mixed greens salad.

Grilled Chicken Breast with Roasted

Squash and Mixed Greens Salad

Description:

This healthy and flavorful meal features grilled chicken breast with roasted squash and a mixed greens salad. The chicken is marinated in a tangy and slightly sweet marinade before being grilled to perfection, while the squash is roasted until tender and caramelized. The mixed greens salad adds freshness and crunch to the dish.

Ingredients:

- 2 boneless, skinless chicken breasts
- 2 cups cubed butternut squash
- 1 tablespoon olive oil
- 1 tablespoon honey
- 1 tablespoon Dijon mustard
- 1 tablespoon apple cider vinegar
- Salt and pepper, to taste
- 4 cups mixed greens
- 1/2 cup cherry tomatoes, halved
- 1/4 cup sliced red onion
- 1/4 cup crumbled feta cheese

Instructions:

1. Preheat grill to medium-high heat.

2. In a small bowl, whisk together the olive oil, honey, Dijon mustard, apple cider vinegar, salt, and pepper.

3. Add the chicken breasts to a large resealable bag and pour the marinade over them. Seal the bag and massage the marinade into the chicken to evenly coat. Let marinate in the refrigerator for at least 30 minutes.

4. Meanwhile, preheat the oven to 400°F. Toss the cubed squash with olive oil, salt, and pepper and spread it out in a single layer on a baking sheet. Roast for 20-25 minutes, until tender and caramelized.

5. Remove the chicken from the marinade and grill for 6-8 minutes per side, or until the internal temperature reaches 165°F.

6. In a large bowl, combine the mixed greens, cherry tomatoes, red onion, and feta cheese. Toss with your favorite dressing.

7. Serve the grilled chicken breast with the roasted squash and mixed greens salad on the side.

Nutritional Information:

- Calories: 380

- Fat: 15g
- Carbohydrates: 29g
- Fiber: 5g

- Protein: 34g

Vegetable and Black Bean Enchiladas with Brown Rice

Description:

This vegetarian meal is loaded with flavorful veggies and black beans, wrapped in tortillas and smothered in enchilada sauce, and served with a side of brown rice. It's a satisfying and healthy dinner option that's perfect for a cozy night in.

Ingredients:

- 8 whole wheat tortillas
- 1 tablespoon olive oil
- 1 small onion, diced
- 1 red bell pepper, diced
- 1 green bell pepper, diced
- 2 garlic cloves, minced

- 1 teaspoon ground cumin
- 1 teaspoon chili powder
- 1 can black beans, drained and rinsed
- 1 cup frozen corn
- 1 cup enchilada sauce
- 1/2 cup shredded cheddar cheese
- Salt and pepper, to taste
- 2 cups cooked brown rice

Instructions:

1. Preheat oven to 375°F.

2. In a large skillet, heat the olive oil over medium-high heat. Add the onion and bell peppers and cook until they begin to soften, about 5 minutes.

3. Add the garlic, cumin, chili powder, black beans, and frozen corn to the skillet. Stir to combine and cook for an additional 2-3 minutes.

4. Grease a 9x13 inch baking dish with cooking spray. Spread a spoonful of enchilada sauce on the bottom of the dish.

5. Warm the tortillas in the microwave or oven to make them more pliable.

6. Spoon the vegetable and black bean mixture onto each tortilla, rolling them up tightly and

placing them seam-side down in the baking dish.

7. Pour the remaining enchilada sauce over the tortillas, spreading it evenly. Sprinkle the shredded cheese over the top.

8. Bake in the preheated oven for 20-25 minutes, until the cheese is melted and bubbly.

9. Serve the enchiladas with a side of brown rice.

Nutritional Information:

- Calories: 410
- Fat: 11g
- Carbohydrates: 67g
- Fiber: 13g
- Protein: 17g

Roasted Salmon with Mixed Vegetables and Quinoa

Description:

This healthy and delicious meal features roasted salmon, mixed vegetables, and quinoa. The salmon is seasoned with herbs and lemon, while the vegetables are roasted until tender and caramelized. The quinoa adds a satisfying and protein-packed element to the dish.

Ingredients:

- 4 salmon fillets
- 1 tablespoon olive oil
- 1 teaspoon dried thyme
- 1 teaspoon dried rosemary
- 1 lemon, sliced
- Salt and pepper, to taste
- 1 cup mixed vegetables (such as carrots, broccoli, and cauliflower), chopped into bite-sized pieces
- 1 cup cooked quinoa

Instructions:

1. Preheat oven to 400°F.

2. Place the salmon fillets on a baking sheet lined with parchment paper. Drizzle with olive oil and sprinkle with thyme, rosemary, salt, and pepper. Place lemon slices on top of the salmon.

3. Toss the mixed vegetables with olive oil, salt, and pepper. Spread them out on a separate baking sheet.

4. Roast the salmon and vegetables in the preheated oven for 15-20 minutes, or until the

salmon is cooked through and the vegetables are tender and caramelized.

5. Serve the salmon and mixed vegetables over a bed of cooked quinoa.

Nutritional Information:

- Calories: 425
- Fat: 18g
- Carbohydrates: 30g
- Fiber: 6g
- Protein: 34g

Grilled Portobello Mushroom Cap Stuffed with Quinoa and Mixed Vegetables

Description:

This vegetarian dish is packed with flavor and nutrition. Grilled portobello mushroom caps are filled with a hearty mixture of quinoa and mixed vegetables, making for a satisfying and delicious meal.

Ingredients:

- 4 large portobello mushroom caps
- 2 tablespoons olive oil

- Salt and pepper, to taste

- 1 cup cooked quinoa

- 1 cup mixed vegetables (such as zucchini, bell peppers, and onions), chopped into bite-sized pieces

- 1 garlic clove, minced

- 1/4 cup fresh parsley, chopped

- 1/4 cup feta cheese, crumbled

Instructions:

1. Preheat a grill to medium-high heat.

2. Brush the mushroom caps with olive oil and sprinkle with salt and pepper.

3. Grill the mushroom caps for 5-7 minutes on each side, or until tender and lightly charred.

4. In a separate pan, sauté the mixed vegetables and garlic in olive oil until tender.

5. Stir in the cooked quinoa, parsley, and feta cheese, and cook for an additional 2-3 minutes, until heated through.

6. Spoon the quinoa and vegetable mixture into the grilled mushroom caps.

7. Return the stuffed mushroom caps to the grill and cook for an additional 2-3 minutes, until heated through.

Nutritional Information:

- Calories: 180
- Fat: 9g
- Carbohydrates: 20g
- Fiber: 5g
- Protein: 8g

Turkey and Vegetable Stir-Fry with Brown Rice

Description:

This stir-fry is a healthy and flavorful way to enjoy lean protein and plenty of colorful vegetables. Served over brown rice, it's a satisfying meal that will leave you feeling nourished and energized.

Ingredients:

- 1 pound ground turkey
- 2 tablespoons olive oil
- 2 garlic cloves, minced
- 1 tablespoon fresh ginger, minced
- 1 onion, chopped
- 1 bell pepper, sliced
- 1 zucchini, sliced

- 1 cup snow peas
- 2 tablespoons soy sauce
- 1 tablespoon honey
- 1 tablespoon cornstarch
- 1/2 cup chicken or vegetable broth
- 4 cups cooked brown rice

Instructions:

1. Heat 1 tablespoon of olive oil in a large skillet over medium-high heat. Add the ground turkey and cook, stirring occasionally, until browned and cooked through, about 8-10 minutes. Remove the turkey from the skillet and set aside.

2. In the same skillet, heat the remaining tablespoon of olive oil over medium-high heat. Add the garlic and ginger and cook for 1-2 minutes, until fragrant.

3. Add the onion, bell pepper, zucchini, and snow peas to the skillet and cook for 5-7 minutes, stirring occasionally, until the vegetables are tender-crisp.

4. In a small bowl, whisk together the soy sauce, honey, cornstarch, and chicken or vegetable broth until smooth.

5. Return the turkey to the skillet and pour the soy sauce mixture over the turkey and

vegetables. Stir to combine.

6. Cook for an additional 2-3 minutes, until the sauce has thickened and the turkey and vegetables are evenly coated.

7. Serve the stir-fry over cooked brown rice.

Nutritional Information:

- Calories: 380
- Fat: 12g
- Carbohydrates: 43g
- Fiber: 5g
- Protein: 25g

CONCLUSION

The Endomorph Diet is a dietary approach designed for individuals with a specific body type called endomorphs. Endomorphs are those who have a naturally higher body fat percentage and a slower metabolism compared to other body types. The Endomorph Diet focuses on macronutrient balance, caloric intake, and regular exercise to help individuals lose weight and improve their overall health.

9 798387 954764